HEALTHY AND HAPPY

DESPITE DIABETES:

Know it, live, and be happy.

TRACE MORGAN

TABLE OF CONTENTS

INTRODUCTION

The chronic disease diabetes, which changes the way the body uses glucose (blood sugar), highlights the important link between diet and general wellbeing. Correct treatment of diabetes depends on a healthy, well-balanced diet. Combining conscious living strategies, including regular exercise and stress management, will help people's quality of life be much better and lower their risk of diabetes-related issues. Apart from balancing blood sugar, this all-encompassing approach promotes longevity and general wellness. Diabetes is today viewed as a strong agent for basic personal transformation. Apart from its physical challenges, diabetes calls for a whole approach that changes relationships, attitudes, and ways of life. Those with this disease must adopt healthy habits, grow resilient, and apply preventative healthcare

Managing diabetes requires tracking blood sugar levels, changing to a nutritious diet, frequent exercise, and occasionally insulin or prescription use. Unchecked diabetes can cause major problems compromising the kidneys, blood vessels, nerves, heart, and eyes. Maintaining good health and avoiding complications depend critically on early diagnosis and appropriate treatment.

CHAPTER ONE

What is Diabetes?

Diabetes is a continual situation resulting from both inadequate insulin manufacturing through the pancreas or abnormal insulin usage through the body.

Insulin is a hormone generated by beta cells in the pancreas that regulates blood sugar (glucose) levels. Insulin is secreted when blood glucose levels rise, such as after a meal. When blood glucose levels fall, insulin secretion stops, and the liver releases glucose into the bloodstream.

Hyperglycemia, commonly known as elevated blood glucose or blood sugar, is a common complication of untreated diabetes that causes catastrophic damage to many of the body's systems, particularly the neurons and blood vessels. Glucose is the body's number one supply of energy. Your body can produce glucose, but it also comes from the foods you eat. Insulin is a pancreatic hormone that facilitates the transport of glucose into cells for use as energy. If you have diabetes, your frame both does no longer produce sufficient insulin or does no longer use it efficiently. Glucose then stays on your stream and no longer attains your cells.

Diabetes increases the risk of vision, kidney, nerve, and heart disease. Diabetes is also connected to certain types of cancer. Taking actions to prevent or manage diabetes can reduce your risk of having diabetes-related health issues.

Types of Diabetes:

There are several types of diabetes, but we will talk about type 1, type 2, and gestational diabetes.

Type 1 diabetes

Often known as juvenile diabetes, it develops when the body fails to manufacture insulin. Insulin is a hormone that breaks down blood sugar and distributes it throughout the body. An individual with type 1 diabetes may also be diagnosed as early as childhood. People with kind 1 diabetes should often take insulin. Individuals can acquire this through injections or an insulin pump. There isn't any therapy for type 1 diabetes. Once diagnosed, they should periodically take a look at their blood sugar levels, provide insulin, and enforce a few lifestyle modifications to help control the illness. Successful blood sugar management can help people with type 1 diabetes avoid serious consequences. If you have type 1 diabetes, your body produces little to no insulin. Your immune system assaults and destroys the cells on your pancreas that produce insulin.

Type 1 diabetes is commonly recognized in youngsters and younger adults, however it may increase at any age.

People with type 1 diabetes need to take insulin each day to live.

Type 2 diabetes:

Type 2 diabetes produces elevated blood sugar levels. Type 2 diabetes can develop gradually, with minor symptoms in the beginning. As a result, many people may not be aware that they have this illness. Type 2 diabetes produces elevated blood sugar levels.

Increased thirst, frequent urination, and weariness are early indications of type 2 diabetes. Type 2 diabetes can develop gradually, with minor symptoms in the beginning. As a result, many people may not be aware that they have this illness.

Early indications and symptoms of type 2 diabetes may include:

Frequent urination:

When blood sugar levels are high, the kidneys try to get rid of the extra sugar via means of filtering it from the blood. This can result in a person needing to urinate more frequently, especially at night.

Increased thirst:

The common urine required to do away with extra sugar from the blood can cause the body to lose extra water. Over time, this could result in dehydration and improved thirst.

Frequent hunger:

People with diabetes often do no longer get sufficient energy from their meals. The digestive tract converts meals right into an easy sugar referred to as glucose, which the body uses as fuel. People with diabetes do no longer get sufficient glucose from the bloodstream into their cells. As a result, people with type 2 diabetes regularly revel

in chronic hunger, no matter the quantity and how frequent they eat.

Fatigue:

Type 2 diabetes can lead to weariness. Diabetes fatigue is due to inadequate sugar flowing from the bloodstream to the body's cells.

Blurry vision:

An overabundance of sugar in the blood can damage the microscopic blood vessels in the eyes, resulting in blurred vision. This can occur in a single or both eyes. High blood glucose levels can also lead to edema of the attention lens. This can cause hazy vision, however it'll enhance as blood sugar levels drop. If a diabetic does not receive treatment, the damage to these blood vessels may worsen, resulting in permanent visual loss.

Slow healing of cuts and wounds:

High blood sugar tiers can lead to nerve and blood vessel damage, impairing blood circulation. As a result, even minor cuts and wounds can also additionally require weeks or months to heal. Slow wound recovery increases the risk of infection.

Tingling, numbness, or soreness on your palms or feet:

High blood sugar levels would possibly disrupt blood stream and damage neurons. In people with type 2 diabetes, this could lead to discomfort, tingling, or numbness of their fingers and feet. This ailment is referred to as neuropathy. If a person does not receive diabetes therapy, their condition may deteriorate over time and lead to more serious consequences.

Patches of dark skin:

Diabetes also can cause darker pores and skin patches to develop within the creases of the neck, armpits, or groin. These areas may feel soft and silky. This pores and skin disease is referred to as acanthosis nigricans.

Itching and yeast infections:

Excess sugar within the blood and urine feeds yeast, which could lead to infection. Warm, moist parts of the skin, such as the mouth, genitals, and armpits, are more prone to yeast infections. The affected areas are normally itchy, but some people feel burning, skin discoloration, and soreness.

Risk Factors for Type 2 Diabetes:

Anyone can get type 2 diabetes; however, certain variables can raise one's risk. These risk factors include: if you are 45 years of age or older, live a sedentary lifestyle, are overweight or obese, consume an imbalanced diet, have a family history of diabetes, have polycystic ovarian syndrome, have a medical history of gestational diabetes, heart disease, or stroke, or have prediabetes, you may be at risk.

Gestational Diabetes:

Gestational diabetes develops during pregnancy as the body becomes less sensitive to insulin. Individuals who are overweight or obese before becoming pregnant are more likely to have the illness. Gestational diabetes may pose some health hazards to both the pregnant woman and the fetus.

These health hazards include the following:

A higher birth weight for the infant, premature birth, low blood sugar levels in the newborn at birth, an increase in the pregnant woman's blood pressure, and an increased risk of the mother developing preeclampsia during pregnancy. Many of the changes associated with gestational diabetes are comparable to those seen during pregnancy. Therefore, there may be no evident signs or symptoms. However, some indications and symptoms include; weariness, impaired eyesight, thirst, nausea, vaginal or skin infections, frequent urination, and urine containing sugar. Any woman who experiences new or odd symptoms while pregnant should consult her doctor. The doctor may be able to detect if she has gestational diabetes or another issue.

Importance of early diagnosis

Since the disease may still be in its early stages and more receptive to treatment, early detection, and treatment can result in better treatment outcomes. Additionally, via means of preventing the disease's development early on and receiving therapy, you'll be able to decrease their danger of growing troubles and beautify their longtime period health.

Taking Care of the Invisible Enemy:

Diabetes is a particularly sneaky disease because it frequently shows no symptoms at the beginning. On the other hand, control measures, including diet, exercise, and medication if needed, can be implemented as a result of an early diagnosis. People can prevent the major issues that come with diabetes by maintaining blood glucose levels within a reasonable range. Therefore, diabetes presents a contradiction in that early detection becomes increasingly crucial the more silent and undetectable the condition is.

Better Results from Treatment:

The best detection is early detection. Individuals who have received a diagnosis can initiate therapies swiftly to correct early-stage problems and avert possibly permanent ones. The need for steeply-priced and volatile procedures is significantly decreased when they are detected early.

Effects of a Late Diagnosis

The Serious Effects on Health:

Diabetes, diagnosed later in life, has serious health effects. The illness may have advanced and resulted in irreversible organ damage by the time symptoms show up and prompt diagnosis. Delays in initiating treatment can aggravate complications such as diabetes retinopathy, neuropathy, and nephropathy.

Healthcare burden on healthcare systems: The delayed diagnosis of diabetes causes problems for the medical community as a whole. Patients frequently require acute care and may need to be hospitalized, which increases management costs. The financial toll affects not just the diagnosed but also undiagnosed people through higher insurance costs. It also extends to hospitals and healthcare providers.

The significance of monitoring your blood sugar.

If you have diabetes, keeping an eye on your glucose levels is essential to determining how well your current treatment plan is working. It provides you with regular and maybe even hourly, guidance on managing your diabetes. When you have diabetes, especially if you need insulin, it's critical to keep an eye on your blood sugar levels. Making decisions about what to eat, how much exercise to do, and how much insulin to take can be aided by the findings of blood sugar monitoring. Numerous factors can impact your blood sugar levels. While some of these effects are extremely difficult or impossible to foresee, you can learn to forecast some of them with time and experience. For this reason, in case your physician advises you to test your blood sugar frequently, it is crucial.

If you have diabetes, you can check your blood sugar at home primarily in two ways: with a finger stick and with an ongoing glucose meter (CGM).

Glucose meter and test strips:

Using a glucose meter and test strips is the most popular method of blood sugar monitoring. This is a "check with a finger stick". To extract a blood drop, you pierce your fingertips with a tiny needle known as a lancet. The glucose meter then displays your blood sugar level in a matter of seconds after you press the drop onto the test strip. People with diabetes, especially those on insulin, frequently need to use finger stick tests multiple times a day because they only measure blood glucose at one specific moment in time.

Constant glucose monitors, or CGMs:

Wearing a device that continuously monitors your blood sugar levels is part of CGM. The gadget creates a graph using this data to provide a more comprehensive view of how your blood sugar levels fluctuate over time. The majority of CGM gadgets employ a small sensor that is inserted beneath your skin. The glucose level in the interstitial fluid, the fluid that exists between your body's cells, is measured by the sensor

What causes your blood sugar to rise?

Taking in carbohydrates, insulin, or diabetic medicine insufficiently, skipping a dose, continuous inactivity or obtaining less exercise than normal, and taking drugs that contain corticosteroids. Stress, illness, or surgery.

The dawn phenomenon is an early morning spike in blood sugar that is probably brought on by hormonal oscillations that occur naturally, such as cortisol, from consuming tobacco. Hydration loss, Adolescence.

Your blood sugar can be lowered by:

losing out on meals. Overdosing on insulin or diabetes medicine.

Movement. Your blood sugar may rise or fall in response to the following circumstances, depending on your biology and other factors: Menstrual cycles or periods. Food and timing of insulin and medications. Consuming alcohol-containing drinks. Drug interactions other than diabetes.

If you have diabetes, it's critical to keep an eye on your blood sugar levels because of these many variables. It's the only way to determine with certainty whether your blood sugar levels are shifting. It also assists you and your healthcare practitioner in understanding how to modify your management.

The function of insulin therapy

Your blood sugar remains within the desired range when on insulin therapy. It assists in averting major issues. To maintain your health if you have type 1 diabetes, you must take insulin therapy. What your body lacks in insulin is replaced by it. Insulin therapy may be included in your care if you have type 2 diabetes. It's necessary if other diabetic therapies and healthy lifestyle modifications aren't controlling your blood sugar levels enough.

Treatment for a kind of diabetes that develops during pregnancy may also occasionally require insulin therapy. Gestational diabetes is the term for this. If good lifestyle choices and other diabetes treatments aren't adequate to control your gestational diabetes, you may require insulin therapy.

CHAPTER TWO

Effect of diabetes on your emotions

Diabetes has an emotional impact in addition to its medical effects. Whether you were just diagnosed or have been living with diabetes for a long time, you may want emotional assistance. This could include stress, depression, or burnout. People around you can sense all of this. Whatever you are experiencing, you're not alone. Living with diabetes can have a major effect on emotional well-being, influencing people differently.

The first diabetes diagnosis could set out;

1. Shock and disbelief:

Accepting the realities of life with a chronic condition usually requires some adjustment. People may experience a range of feelings, from anxiety and hopelessness to uncertainty about what this suggests for their future health.

2. **Anxiety About Management:**

Anxiety can be brought on by worries about long-term difficulties such as nerve damage, kidney disease, or vision problems. Chronic stress can result from daily activities including following food and lifestyle modifications, monitoring blood sugar levels, and giving medications or insulin.

3. **Self-blame and guilt: The Part Played by Lifestyle :**

In type 2 diabetes, when lifestyle factors, including diet and exercise, are crucial, individuals may feel guilty or self-blame for not stopping the condition.

4. **Effect on Self-Esteem:**

These emotions could cause feelings of inadequacy and poor self-esteem.

5. **Emotional suffering and depression:**

Managing diabetes calls for constant attention, which can lead to persistent anxiety. Stress of this kind might cause hopelessness.

Variations in blood sugar levels can produce emotional highs and lows that compromise mood stability, even with the best attempts at control.

6. **Relationships and social dynamics:**

Social Separation: The desire to control food consumption, drugs, and physical exercise can lead to social alienation and cause people to feel different from their friends. Effect on Family and Friends: Loved ones who struggle to understand the requirements of diabetes control may cause conflict or discontent on both sides.

7. **Psychological Impact: Strategies of Coping**

People could create coping mechanisms that include denial, avoidance of diabetes management responsibilities, or an overdependence on unhealthy coping mechanisms, such as comfort eating or drug misuse.

Managing diabetes requires a never-ending emotional rollercoaster of highs and lows, both physically and mentally.

Ways to promote emotional resilience for diabetics

1. Diabetes patients require emotional resilience because managing diabetes presents daily obstacles that may impact their mental health. Here are various techniques to promote emotional resilience:

2. Education and Understanding: Learn about diabetes, how to control it, and the impacts it has. Understanding your situation can

alleviate worry and enable you to make more informed decisions.

3. Build a support network. Surround yourself with people who understand your situation. This can include family members, friends, medical professionals, and support groups. Sharing experiences and receiving support can improve resilience.

4. Healthy Lifestyle Choices: Eat a well-balanced diet, exercise regularly (as prescribed by your doctor), and get enough sleep. These lifestyle choices not only aid with diabetes management but also contribute to general mental well-being.

5. Mindfulness and Stress Management: Use mindfulness practices like meditation, deep

breathing exercises, and yoga. These techniques can help reduce stress, regulate blood pressure, and boost general emotional resilience.

6. Set realistic goals: Break down long-term goals into smaller, more attainable actions. Celebrate your successes along the way, as they can provide motivation and a sense of control over your diabetes management.

7. Seek Professional Help: Don't be afraid to seek help from mental health specialists, such as psychiatrists or counselors. They can offer coping skills, emotional support, and effective stress management approaches. Stay in Touch with Your Healthcare Providers: Discuss your concerns, issues,

and progress with your healthcare team on a regular basis. They can offer advice, check your health, and modify your treatment plan as needed.

8. Manage Negative thoughts: Reframe negative thoughts from a more positive or realistic perspective. This can help to lessen feelings of helplessness and increase overall emotional resilience.

9. Maintain a pattern: Creating a daily pattern that includes regular meals, medication management, and self-care activities can help to provide structure and consistency, which is beneficial for emotional health. Acceptance and Adaptation: Recognize that living with diabetes comprises ups and

downs. Accept the challenges that come your way, and focus on adapting to changes in your health and daily life.

By implementing these tactics into your daily routine, you can improve your emotional resilience as a diabetic and better handle the psychological components of diabetes care. Remember to customize these tactics to meet your specific requirements, and circumstances.

Long life while diabetic? Remember to remain optimistic.

What was life like before diabetes?

If it has been years since your diagnosis, you may find it difficult to remember what it was like before the daily worry about diabetes nutrition, good glucose levels, and care management. Staying positive over time can be difficult, particularly following a setback. It's a lifetime commitment to control your diabetes on a daily basis, and It's Normal to find managing your health demanding. Although it's almost impossible to keep negative ideas away all the time. There are simple everyday techniques you can follow to help you have an overall positive attitude and lead a happy, fulfilled life.

1. One should celebrate the small things.

Your diabetic journey may seem drawn out. Emphasizing successes in the little moments will help one grow positively.

For one day, for instance, try to test your blood sugar as advised by your doctor. When you succeed, credit yourself. Expanding on that achievement, try to do it tomorrow. Better yet, use continuous glucose monitoring to collaborate with your healthcare provider to identify simpler methods for maintaining satisfactory glucose levels.

2. Simplify personal management:

Although you will always have to manage your condition, following the most recent developments in diabetes treatment will help you make it easier. An important component of the diabetes diet is tracking your progress and monitoring your glucose levels, but it can take a lot of time and effort. Luckily, life-changing technologies can make diabetes self-management easier.

For instance, the Freestyle Libre system is a continuous glucose monitoring device. It automatically measures and logs glucose readings for up to ten days, eliminating the need for finger sticks. Talk to your doctor about whether updating your management schedule or technology may be a suitable fit for you.

3. Tune up your eating plan.

Spend some time on diabetes nutrition by looking at your daily dietary choices. If you find yourself bored with your diet, vary it to make mealtimes exciting once more. Research new recipes to try or try adjusting your favorite ones to be diabetic-friendly. Use several seasonings to keep things interesting.

Still another concept: snack wisely. Snacks are an excellent way to fit in a fruit or vegetable portion and provide a diversity of textures to your diet. Options can be a sweet potato you bake and top with cinnamon or use to create your own baked potato chips or quinoa and blueberry salad. Another excellent option is unsalted nuts. Keep your blood glucose levels under control.

4. Turn negative ideas around.

Be conscious of your ideas. Whenever you notice yourself thinking negatively, translate that adverse notion into a positive statement. Here are tips:

If you find yourself saying, "I can't do this anymore," rethink as, "I am strong. I am capable of this!

Instead of, "I ate a big slice of cake at the celebration. Tell yourself, "Okay, so I didn't completely follow my eating plan today, but I eat so much better than I used to. I blew it again. At my next meal, I will be quickly back on track.

Swap "I'm uninterested in combating diabetes," for "I'm operating to stay my best, fullest existence possible. Don't punish yourself for not being flawless. Positive self-talk can significantly change your viewpoint.

5. Pursue your love projects.

Discover something that brings you joy, and schedule daily time even just fifteen minutes to engage in it. Your activities can be reading a book, meditating, walking your dog, painting, or learning a musical instrument.

Schedule daily time for whatever makes you happy, and rank it among your priorities. Spending this time for fun can help you live a balanced, healthy life and think positively.

6. Emphasize your areas of control.

Constantly worrying about the things you cannot control can easily become a habit. Remind yourself that diabetes care is only one aspect of your life; you are in charge of your actions, not the diabetes, thus, try to keep things in perspective.

Pay attention to what you can influence, including your diet, workout schedule, treatment options, and doctors. Remember that every good deed helps to reduce your future chances of problems.

7. Connect with others.

No matter how long you have had diabetes, it is never too late to enjoy the advantages of socializing with people on the same path.

CHAPTER THREE

Diabetes management and prevention

Diabetes is a condition caused by one's lifestyle. Changing your lifestyle will eliminate those conditions. Just be careful with what you consume and imagine how much better your blood sugar will be next time.

Diabetes can be prevented and controlled in several ways. This comprises;

Choosing a healthy lifestyle:

You may stop smoking, manage your weight through good eating and exercise, discover constructive ways to cope with stress and avoid or delay the onset of diabetes or its effects on your body. Maintaining a healthy lifestyle will also lower your chance of getting additional illnesses.

Know your numbers:

You can check your blood sugar, blood pressure, blood cholesterol, and weight at home and during routine appointments with your healthcare team. These vital health indicators give you a sense of how effectively your diabetes treatment plan is managing your condition and preserving your general health.

Collaborate with your medical team.

Diabetes may impact your heart, legs, feet, and vision. It may also call for certain diet and drug regimens. As a result, your healthcare team could consist of several specialists from different fields of medicine. Your team can help you reduce the impacts of diabetes on your body by guiding you through your treatment plan.

Wholesome eating practices whether you have type 1 or type 2 diabetes, you may want to hold your present-day weight or lessen it. However, even as you are doing this, it is important to pick healthful foods.

Healthy eating habits

Generally, it's good to eat healthy even when you don't have any illness. Developing healthy eating habits is essential for maintaining overall wellbeing not just for diabetics alone.

Healthy eating will help you make the right choices of food to consume while minding your portion size.

Managing your glucose level involves making informed food choices, maintaining consistency and being careful on how those foods impact your blood sugar level. In some cases, it's good to work with a registered dietitian. Healthy foods when battling with diabetes helps you a lot.

Here are some tips:

- **Select more nutritious carbs.**

Knowing which meals include carbohydrates is vital due to the fact all of them affect blood glucose levels. Pick the extra nutritious meals that might be excessive in carbohydrates, and watch how much you eat. These are a few nutritious places to get carbohydrates: entire grains like buckwheat, brown rice, and whole oats; fruits; vegetables; pulses like lentils, beans, and chickpeas; dairy products like milk and yogurt without added sugar. Reducing your intake of low-fiber foods like white bread, white rice, and highly processed cereal is also crucial.

- **Consume less salt.**

Consuming a high-salt diet can raise your blood pressure, which raises your risk of heart disease and stroke. Furthermore, all of those ailments already include an improved threat when you have diabetes. Aim to consume no more than 6 g (one teaspoon) of salt each day. Many pre-packaged foods already have salt in them, so make sure to examine meal labels and pick objects with decreased salt content. Making food from scratch will permit you to screen your salt intake.

- **Reduce your intake of processed and red meat.**

You may also discover that you want to devour large servings of meat to be full while you are cutting back on carbohydrates. However, the usage of red and processed meats, together with ham, bacon, sausages, cattle, and lamb, in this manner isn't recommended. These are all related to most cancers and coronary heart issues. Consider replacing processed and red meat with these: pulses like lentils and beans, eggs Fish, poultry, such as turkey and chicken, unsalted almonds, Beans, peas, and lentils are excellent options to processed and beef for the reason that they're low in blood sugar and excessive in fiber, at the same time as additionally supporting you feel full. Better still are oily fish, such as mackerel and salmon. They contain a lot of omega-3 oil, which supports heart health.

- **Consume more veggies and fruits.**

You may maintain your health by consuming a diet high in fruits and vegetables, as they provide your body with the necessary vitamins, minerals, and fiber. Choose the entire fruit whenever possible, as fruit liquids include sugar that is considered free sugar. This may be canned (in juice, no longer syrup), dried, frozen, or fresh.

Additionally, eating small portions throughout the day is preferable to eating a larger one at once.

- **Choose healthier fats**

Nuts, seeds, avocados, oily seafood, olive oil, rapeseed oil, and sunflower oil are all foods high in healthy fats.

- **Reduce your intake of free sugar**

We all know that giving up sugar can be pretty tough at first, so making modest, achievable adjustments is a clever area to begin while trying to lessen your intake of added sugar.

Replace sugar-stuffed beverages, fruit juices, and energy drinks with sugar-unfastened water, simple milk, tea, and coffee. Eliminating free sugar can help you control your weight and blood glucose levels.

To assist you lessen lower back pain, you could constantly strive for low- or zero-calorie sweeteners (on occasion known as synthetic or non-sugar sweeteners). In the fast run, these also can lead to weight reduction in case you do not replace them with different high-calorie meals and beverages.

However, over time, take some time to reduce all sorts of sweetness on your diet.

- **Use your snacks wisely**

When choosing a snack, avoid chips, cookies, chocolates, and crisps in favor of yogurts, unsalted almonds, seeds, fruits, and vegetables.

- **Consume alcohol in moderation.**

Due to its high-calorie content, alcohol use has to be decreased if weight reduction is your goal. Aim to eat no more than 14 units in a week. However, unfold it out and bypass some days

of alcohol use every week to save you from binge drinking. Drinking on an empty stomach is likewise not a good idea if you use insulin or other diabetes treatments. This is because alcohol may increase the likelihood of hypos.

- **Avoid consuming so-called diabetic foods.**

It is currently illegal to refer to any food as "diabetic food. This is because there is no evidence that consuming those foods will give you unique advantages over eating healthily. They can nonetheless affect your blood glucose level and often have the same quantity of fat and calories as similar foods. Additionally, certain foods occasionally have a laxative effect.

Importance of Sleep for Diabetics

Sleep is critical to people's general health and well-being, especially for diabetics. Here's why diabetics need to sleep and how to get better sleep:

Blood Sugar Control: Adequate sleep helps regulate blood sugar levels by affecting insulin sensitivity and glucose metabolism. Poor sleep can cause insulin resistance, making blood sugar control difficult.

Weight Management: A lack of sleep can affect hormones that regulate hunger and appetite, increasing desires for high-calorie foods. This can lead to weight gain and obesity, both of which are risk factors for diabetes.

Energy Levels and Mood: Getting enough sleep boosts energy and mental clarity, which are essential for sticking to diabetes control routines, including meal planning, exercise, and medication compliance.

Heart Health: Lack of sleep is linked to an increased risk of cardiovascular disease, which is already a concern for many diabetics due to their higher risk of heart problems.

Sleep is crucial for immunological function, poor sleep can weaken the immune system, making diabetics more susceptible to infections and slower to repair wounds.

Tips to Improve Diabetic Sleep Quality

Maintain a Consistent Sleep Schedule: Go to bed and get up at the same time every day, even on weekends. This regulates your body's internal schedule and improves sleep quality.

Set up a relaxing bedtime routine, such as reading, taking a warm bath, or practicing relaxation techniques like deep breathing or meditation. Avoid engaging in stimulating activities or using bright screens close to bedtime.

Create a comfortable sleeping environment. Make your bedroom cool, quiet, and dark. If noise bothers you, use comfortable bedding and think about getting earplugs or a white noise machine.

Limit Stimulants and Alcohol: Avoid consuming caffeine and nicotine close to bedtime because they can disrupt sleep. Limit your alcohol consumption, as it can alter sleep patterns and cause nightly awakenings.

Regular Exercise: Regular physical activity is recommended, but severe exercise should be avoided close to bedtime. Exercise improves sleep quality and can help control blood sugar levels.

Manage stress: Try stress-relieving strategies like yoga, mindfulness, or progressive muscle relaxation. Stress and anxiety can disrupt sleep, so finding techniques to relax before bedtime can be useful.

Limit Fluid Intake Before Bed: Drink less liquid in the evening to reduce overnight bathroom trips, which can disrupt sleep.

Address Sleep Disorders: If you suspect you have a sleep condition, such as sleep apnea or restless legs syndrome, see your doctor for an assessment and treatment. Treating underlying sleep disorders can boost overall sleep quality. Individuals with diabetes can better manage their disease and general health by focusing on excellent sleep hygiene and implementing changes to improve sleep quality. Consistent, restorative sleep is critical for good diabetes treatment and lowering

the risk of complications.

CHAPTER FOUR

Exercise's Benefits for People with Diabetes

Engaging in physical activity is among the best things you can do for your general well-being. For individuals of all ages, engaging in daily physical activity is crucial, as it positively affects both mental and physical health.

Exercise can be beneficial for a diabetic because it improves insulin sensitivity, leads to better diabetes control, lowers blood sugar levels, and lessens insulin resistance. Enhance bone strength and the movement of joints and muscles. Reduce your blood pressure and keep a healthy weight. Lower your chance of developing heart disease. Decrease tension and worry. It helps with a better night's sleep. Because it lowers blood sugar, exercise is essential for managing diabetes.

Importance of exercise for diabetics:

- **Enhances Insulin Sensitivity:** Physical activity makes it easier for your muscles to utilize insulin, which decreases blood sugar.

- **Reduces Blood Sugar Levels:** Exercise has the immediate ability to reduce blood sugar levels and contributes to their long-term stability.

- **Weight control:** Maintaining a healthy weight is crucial for managing type 2 diabetes, and regular exercise can help you reach and maintain it.

- **Enhances Cardiovascular Health:** Exercise strengthens the heart and enhances circulation, whereas diabetes raises the risk of heart disease.

- **Improves All-around Wellness:** Engaging in physical activity helps lower stress levels, elevate mood, and boost vitality, all of which are advantageous for effectively managing diabetes.

- **Type 1 Diabetes Management:** Exercise helps type 1 diabetics lower insulin resistance, improving blood sugar regulation. It's critical to speak with a healthcare professional to identify the ideal kind, amount, and intensity of exercise based on personal health needs and diabetes management objectives if you want to use exercise to control your diabetes.

Types of exercise for diabetics.

People with diabetes can benefit from a variety of exercise modalities. Among them are:

Aerobic Exercise:

Walking, running, cycling, swimming, and dancing are examples of aerobic exercises that enhance cardiovascular health, raise insulin sensitivity, and lower blood sugar. It is advised to perform at least 150 minutes of moderate-intensity aerobic activity per week, ideally over three days, with no more than two days off from the gym in between.

Resistance Exercise:

Building muscle mass through strength training activities like lifting weights or utilizing resistance bands might enhance insulin sensitivity and glucose metabolism. It is advised to incorporate resistance training activities that focus on your primary muscle groups at least twice a week

Exercises for Balance and Flexibility:

Exercises that enhance flexibility, balance, and relaxation, such as tai chi and yoga, can enhance resistance and aerobic training and are beneficial for general health. It is advised that you include flexibility exercises in your regimen on a regular basis, two or three times a week,

Benefits of interval training:

Short bursts of intensive exercise are alternated with rest or lower-intensity activity during interval training. It can be especially useful for raising insulin sensitivity and cardiovascular fitness. It is advised that you incorporate interval training sessions, under the supervision of a fitness expert or healthcare provider, into your aerobic exercise regimen.

Regular Physical Activity:

Even small changes in regular physical activity, like walking short distances instead of driving or using the stairs instead of the elevator, can have a positive impact on blood sugar regulation and general health. Suggestion: Try to move more during the day and cut down on time spent sitting down.

Pre-exercise preparations:

A few essential rules must be followed while designing a safe and efficient workout program for diabetics to guarantee that fitness and health objectives are reached without resulting in issues. Here are some rules to follow:

Talk with a healthcare professional

See your doctor before beginning any workout regimen, particularly if you have diabetes. Personalized advice can be given by them depending on your current state of health.

Selecting the Correct Kind of Exercise

Make sure to choose aerobic, low-impact exercises like cycling, swimming, walking, or dancing.

Engaging in these exercises can help lower blood sugar levels and enhance cardiovascular health.

- **Monitor your blood sugar levels:** To understand how your body reacts to exercise, check your blood sugar levels both before and after. This assists in modifying your regimen to avoid hypoglycemia or low blood sugar.

- **Stay Hydrated:** To avoid dehydration, which can impact blood sugar levels, drink lots of water before, during, and after exercise.

- **Progressively Boost Intensity:** As your fitness level rises, start with low intensity workouts and gradually increase the time and intensity over time. This method aids in preventing abrupt increases or decreases in blood sugar levels.

- **Include Strength Training:** To increase muscle strength, perform resistance training activities with weights or resistance bands. More efficient glucose utilization by muscle tissue can aid in blood sugar regulation.

- **Warm-up and cool-down:** To get your body ready for activity and help with recuperation, always start with a warm-up and finish with a cool-down.

- **Wear the correct footwear:** People with diabetes need to take greater care of their feet. Make sure your shoes fit properly and are comfortable, and check your feet frequently for any signs of damage.

- **Bring Snacks:** When exercising, carry fruit juice, glucose pills, or other fast-acting carbs in case your blood sugar drops suddenly.

- **Pay Attention to Your Body:** If you feel weak or dizzy, or if you experience any other unusual symptoms, stop exercising immediately. This can be a sign that something is wrong with your blood sugar levels.

Be careful when exercising if you have diabetes, if you are feeling sick or have ketones in your blood or urine, avoid engaging in vigorous physical activity. Make sure you drink enough water before, during, and after physical activity.

CHAPTER FIVE

Live and be happy

Living well with diabetes involves not only managing blood sugar levels but also maintaining overall well-being and happiness.

Whatever you are experiencing, you're not alone, never ever allow negative thoughts, you can always be happy and healthy despite being sick. All you need is to improve yourself.

Being diagnosed with diabetes is not the end of one's life, it will surely get better when you improve your lifestyle. You can do this! Get up and Go.

If you find yourself saying, "I can't do this anymore," rethink as, "I am strong. I am capable of this!

Instead of, "I ate a big slice of cake at the celebration. Tell yourself, "Okay, so I didn't completely follow my eating plan today, but I eat so much better than I used to. I blew it again. At my next meal, I will be quickly back on track.

Swap "I'm uninterested in combating diabetes," for "I'm operating to stay my best, fullest existence possible. Don't punish yourself for not being flawless. Positive self-talk can significantly change your viewpoint.

Know your sick-day rules, and attend appointments as directed by your healthcare team.

To maintain good health, keep critical numbers ready, prioritize physical activity, get enough sleep, and wash your hands frequently.

If you're staying at home, make sure to care for your mental health. Maintain contact with loved ones, say no to unnecessary commitments, and seek assistance as needed. It is critical to inform your family and friends about the hardships of living with diabetes.

Sleep is essential for preserving bodily and intellectual health. Many diabetics develop sleep disturbances. If you believe your sleep is interfering with your life, schedule an appointment with your doctor right away.

Being involved in a community can improve your mental health. Walking with a friend, joining an exercise group, eating with others, or becoming a regular at your neighborhood coffee shop can all help to make life feel more meaningful. Volunteering has also been found to offer tremendous health advantages!

Diabetes is like a roller coaster, with ups and downs; motivation is what gets you going.

Diabetes is a condition caused by one's lifestyle, changing your lifestyle will eliminate those conditions. Just be careful with what you consume.

Just imagine how much better your blood sugar will be next time.

Never worry about it, live and be happy.

You will be alright.